ROTATOR CUFF SURGERY DIET

Transformative Nutrition Strategies And Nourishing Recovery For Muscle And Shoulder Joint

DR LUCAS KAYCE

DISCLAIMER

This book about illness and nutrition is not meant to replace expert medical advice, diagnosis, or treatment; rather, it is meant purely for informational reasons. This book's content is founded on broad concepts and recommendations for managing diseases and nutrition.

Before adopting any major dietary or lifestyle changes, readers are recommended to speak with a qualified healthcare provider, such as a licensed physician or registered dietitian, especially if they have pre-existing medical concerns. Everybody has different health demands, so what works for one person might not work for another.

The use of the information provided in this book may have unfavorable repercussions or consequences, for which the author and publisher disclaim all liability. No disease is meant to be identified, treated, cured, or prevented by the information provided.

The book may include contain references to medical literature or research findings; however readers are urged to independently confirm this material and contact reliable sources.

It is important to remember that the fields of nutrition and medicine are always changing, and that new findings could have an impact on the advice offered in this book. As a result, readers are urged to keep up with the most recent advancements in healthcare and, when in doubt, seek professional counsel.

By reading this book, readers agree that they are in charge of their own health decisions and release the author and publisher from any liability arising from the use of the material in the book, whether direct or indirect.

TABLE OF CONTENTS

ABOUT THE BOOK

A crucial component of the healing process after rotator cuff surgery is the significance of nutrition, which is covered in the book "Rotator Cuff Surgery Diet". The book begins with a thorough review of rotator cuff surgery, highlighting the role that a well-planned diet plays in the recovery process. This introduction lays the groundwork for readers to comprehend the role that diet plays in the healing process following surgery.

The book covers the basic principles of rotator cuff surgery, including information on the structure of the rotator cuff, typical injury sources, surgical indications, and preoperative measures. This background information creates a framework in which readers can understand the complexities of the healing process.

The book then turns to the importance of nutrition in the healing phase, examining how nutrition affects inflammation and healing as well as the particular nutrients needed for tissue repair.

The dietary recommendations made in the following chapters have a strong justification in this chapter.

The book discusses the how-to of putting a post-surgery diet into practice. Readers receive instructions on how to set up their kitchens, follow post-surgery dietary guidelines, and use supplements to aid in their recuperation. Assisting patients after rotator cuff surgery with their immediate and long-term nutritional demands, sample meal plans, and hydration techniques are offered.

The relationship between nutrition and exercise is highlighted, which also explains how physical therapy and exercise can be incorporated gradually into the healing process. This all-encompassing method recognizes the mutual benefits of diet and recovery.

It concludes the subject by addressing long-term issues, advising readers to lead healthy lifestyles, discussing nutrition for joint health, and providing advice on how to avoid being hurt again. This thorough handbook helps people not just in the short term during their recovery but also gives them the knowledge they need to continue living a healthy lifestyle once their rehabilitation is complete.

"Rotator Cuff Surgery Diet" is essentially an invaluable tool for anyone having rotator cuff surgery since it emphasizes the critical role that nutrition plays in the healing process and provides a comprehensive approach to rehabilitation. The book's well-organized content guarantees that readers will get helpful advice supported by a thorough comprehension of the surgical process and its ramifications.

CHAPTER ONE

ROTATOR CUFF SURGERY DIET OVERVIEW

OVERVIEW OF SURGERY ON THE ROTATOR CUFF

A medical technique called rotator cuff surgery is used to treat problems involving the rotator cuff, which is a collection of tendons and muscles that surround the shoulder joint. These vital structures are essential for promoting stability and range of motion in the shoulder. People who have rotator cuff damage may have shoulder pain, weakness, and restricted range of motion.

This damage can result from an injury, degeneration, or other circumstances. The goal of rotator cuff surgery is to relieve symptoms and restore functionality by reconstructing or repairing these injured structures.

The degree and kind of the injury will determine the surgical methods used in rotator cuff surgery.

Depending on the patient's needs, common operations include tendon transfers, open repairs, and arthroscopic repairs. Little incisions are made during arthroscopy, a minimally invasive procedure that uses a camera to direct the surgeon and shortens recovery times and postoperative pain. Conversely, open repairs need a bigger incision and provide the surgeon with a clear view of the injured tissues. When there is a great loss of tissue and the neighboring tendons need to be realigned to restore function, tendon transplants may be an option.

Following rotator cuff surgery, recovery is a complex process that includes physical therapy, rehabilitation exercises, and following postoperative care guidelines. Rebuilding strength and flexibility are essential for a full recovery, therefore the patient's commitment to rehabilitation is typically a determining factor in the success of the surgery. Patients who are having rotator cuff surgery should be realistic about how long they will need to recuperate and realize that it could take weeks or months to get back to their regular activities.

DIET IS CRUCIAL TO THE HEALING PROCESS

Although surgery is a crucial step in treating rotator cuff problems, nutrition plays a significant role in the healing process and should not be undervalued. A vital component of postoperative treatment, nutrition plays a critical role in the body's capacity to recover and regenerate tissues. Sufficient nutritional intake can speed up the healing process and improve the overall outcome of the procedure.

As the basic building unit of tissues, protein is especially important during the healing stage. By encouraging the production of collagen, a protein essential to the integrity of connective tissues, it helps heal injured muscles and tendons. Incorporating lean protein sources, like fish, chicken, beans, and tofu, into the postoperative diet can aid in tissue recovery.

A balanced diet full of vitamins and minerals is just as important as protein. Minerals like calcium and phosphorus affect bone strength, whereas vitamins like C and D support collagen formation and bone health, respectively. The right nutrients can be obtained for optimum recuperation with a diet rich in whole grains, dairy products, fruits, and vegetables.

Another essential component of postoperative treatment is hydration. Maintaining adequate hydration promotes healthy bodily functioning, facilitates the movement of nutrients, and aids in the removal of pollutants from the body. To speed up the healing process, people recovering from rotator cuff surgery should make drinking enough water a priority.

A well-balanced, nutrient-rich diet combined with rotator cuff surgery can greatly accelerate the healing process. Comprehending the complexities of both facets enables individuals to take a comprehensive approach to their rehabilitation, so facilitating the healing of the surgical site as well as the patient's general well-being.

CHAPTER TWO

COMPREHENDING SURGERY ON THE ROTATOR CUFF

THE ROTATOR CUFF ANATOMY

A vital collection of tendons and muscles that envelop the shoulder joint and offer stability and a broad range of motion is known as the rotator cuff. The rotator cuff, which is made up of the teres minor, subscapularis, supraspinatus, and infraspinatus muscles, is essential to the healthy operation of the shoulder. Together, these muscles enable the arm to be raised, extended, and rotated. A cuff that holds the shoulder joint together is formed by the rotator cuff's tendons attaching to the head of the humerus.

TYPICAL REASONS FOR INJURIES TO THE ROTATOR CUFF

Injuries to the rotator cuff are frequent and can have several causes. These injuries can result from a variety of sources, including trauma, aging, overuse, and degeneration. In sports like baseball or tennis, repetitive overhead motions can cause the rotator cuff to gradually deteriorate over time. Acute injuries like rotator cuff strains or tears can also result from abrupt, violent motions or direct impact on the shoulder.

REASONS TO HAVE A ROTATOR CUFF SURGERY

Surgery might be required if non-invasive measures like physical therapy, anti-inflammatory drugs, and rest don't work to relieve the symptoms of a rotator cuff injury. Prolonged pain, weakness, and functional restrictions that affect everyday activities and quality of life are indications for rotator cuff surgery. Imaging tests, such as magnetic resonance imaging (MRI) scans, assist physicians in selecting the best course of action by evaluating the kind and extent of rotator cuff injury.

GETTING READY FOR SURGERY

The orthopedic surgeon will perform a comprehensive evaluation to prepare you for rotator cuff surgery.

Preoperative evaluations of patients may involve physical examinations, extra diagnostic testing, and reviews of their medical histories to make sure they are a good fit for surgery. It is crucial to let the surgical team know about any underlying medical issues, allergies, or prescriptions. In addition, patients are recommended to stop taking several drugs, such as blood thinners, in the days preceding surgery to reduce the possibility of bleeding issues during the process.

Patients receive education regarding the surgical process, possible risks, and anticipated results during the preoperative phase. Before surgery, prehabilitation activities are frequently advised to maximize shoulder function and strength. The patient and the medical staff need to communicate clearly to address any concerns and guarantee a seamless transition into the operation room. The effectiveness of rotator cuff surgery and the recovery period that follows are greatly influenced by the cooperative work of the patient and the surgical team during the preparatory phase.

CHAPTER THREE

THE DIET'S FUNCTION IN HEALING

NUTRITION'S CRUCIAL ROLE IN HEALING

It is impossible to exaggerate the impact that nutrition plays in the healing process because it is essential to the body's natural healing processes. A nutritious and well-balanced diet is critical for supplying the necessary nutrients that support tissue regeneration and repair, enabling people to recover from disease, trauma, or surgery. Inadequate dietary support might jeopardize the healing process, causing problems and healing delays.

THE IMPACT OF FOOD ON INFLAMMATION

The influence of diet on inflammation is a crucial component of the link between nutrition and healing. While some degree of inflammation is normal and essential for the healing process, persistent or extreme inflammation can hinder healing and lead to consequences.

Certain dietary decisions have the potential to exacerbate or lessen inflammation. Antioxidant-rich diets that include whole grains, fruits, and vegetables have been demonstrated to have anti-inflammatory properties that help control inflammation and promote healing.

ESSENTIAL NUTRIENTS FOR REPAIRING TISSUE

Numerous nutrients are essential for tissue regeneration and repair. For example, proteins are necessary building blocks for the synthesis of new proteins and the healing of damaged tissues.

Sufficient consumption of protein is especially crucial for those recuperating from operations or accidents because it promotes the synthesis of collagen and other structural elements required for tissue repair.

In addition, some biochemical pathways involved in wound healing and tissue repair depend on vitamins and minerals such as copper, zinc, vitamin E, and vitamin C.

HYDRATION AND HOW IT AFFECTS HEALING

Another crucial element that has a big impact on the healing process is hydration. Sustaining cellular activity and preserving the body's general functionality depends on enough hydration.

Water is essential for many physiological functions, such as waste removal, temperature regulation, and nutrition transfer. People may require more fluids while recovering from an illness because of things like fever, perspiration, or higher metabolic demands. Dehydration can interfere with these functions and make it more difficult for the body to recover itself.

Nutrition plays a complex role in recovery and includes things like how important it is to heal, how diet affects inflammation, what nutrients are necessary for tissue regeneration, and how important it is to stay hydrated.

During difficult times of sickness, accident, or surgery, a thoughtful and well-balanced approach to nutrition can maximize the body's healing processes, enhance recovery results, and contribute to general well-being.

CHAPTER FOUR

GETTING YOUR KITCHEN READY

PURCHASING NUTRIENT-RICH FOODS IN BULK

A carefully stocked pantry and refrigerator are the foundation of every well-prepared kitchen. Make nutrient-rich foods a priority to make sure your meals not only satisfy you but also improve your general health. Add a range of fresh produce, whole grains, lean meats, dairy products, and plant-based substitutes. For a variety of nutrients, try including foods like legumes, brown rice, quinoa, nuts, and seeds. Aim for a mix of macronutrients, including fats, proteins, and carbohydrates, to help your body meet its energy requirements and perform vital tasks.

To have easy substitutes on hand, use canned or frozen fruits and vegetables in addition to fresh products. Lentils, chickpeas, and canned beans are great plant-based protein sources that are simple to include in a variety of recipes.

Nuts, avocados, and olive oil are good sources of healthy fats that can improve the flavor and nutritional value of your food. To enhance fiber consumption and support digestive health, go for whole-grain versions of essential foods like bread, pasta, and cereals.

APPLIANCES & KITCHEN TOOLS FOR SIMPLE MEAL PREPARATION

Having the proper kitchenware and appliances tremendously facilitates efficient meal preparation. To ensure a flawless culinary experience, spend money on top-notch chopping and slicing blades, cutting boards, and mixing bowls. While stainless steel pans are robust and adaptable, non-stick cookware can simplify cooking and cleanup. To manage various cooking procedures, think about keeping a range of utensils on hand, such as ladles, tongs, and spatulas.

Time-saving and versatile culinary tools such as a food processor, blender, and slow cooker are made of little but powerful parts. Precise ingredient measurements are ensured with a sturdy set of measuring cups and spoons, particularly when following instructions. When you are motivated to bake, stock your kitchen with baking pans, rolling pins, and sheets. A kitchen that is neatly arranged, with specific areas for every appliance, can expedite the cooking process and enhance the overall gastronomic delight.

ORGANIZING AND CREATING A MENU

Efficient meal planning and arrangement are fundamental elements of a properly equipped kitchen. Start by putting together a weekly or monthly meal plan with a range of recipes, accounting for various food categories and dietary needs. This makes food shopping easier and helps to guarantee a balanced diet. To cut down on wasteful spending and minimize food waste, think about creating a shopping list that is based on your meal plan.

Methodically arrange your kitchen, keeping commonly used goods close at hand. Organize your refrigerator and pantry so that you can find ingredients easily when preparing meals.

To keep perishables fresh, think about utilizing storage containers that are clearly labeled for simple identification. Every week, set aside time to prepare meals. This can include chopping vegetables, marinating proteins, or making ingredients that can be used in a variety of recipes. By taking the initiative, you can make healthy eating more accessible and save time on hectic days.

Having the proper kitchenware, organizing and planning meals efficiently, and storing up nutrient-dense foods are all essential components of a well-prepared kitchen. You can facilitate healthy eating, make meal preparation easier, and improve your whole cooking experience by concentrating on these ideas.

CHAPTER FIVE

RIGHT AFTER SURGERY DIET

To aid in the healing process and advance general recovery following surgery, post-surgical nutrition must be carefully considered. To maximize potential consequences and guarantee that patients get the nutrients they need, the immediate post-surgery diet is essential. A clear liquid diet is frequently advised at first to help the digestive system gradually return to normal. During this stage, easily digested liquids including water, clear juices, and broth are usually consumed. Providing vital electrolytes and avoiding dehydration are the main priorities at this time.

MAKING THE SWITCH TO SOFT FOODS

Patients frequently move from a clear liquid diet to soft meals as their recuperation advances. By introducing solid foods gradually, the risk of postoperative problems is reduced while the digestive system adjusts. The easily chewable and digested texture of soft foods makes them kinder on the recovering gastrointestinal tract. Yogurt, mashed potatoes, and pureed veggies are a few examples of soft foods. This phase makes sure the surgical site isn't overworked while yet providing patients with enough nourishment.

INTRODUCING SOLID FOODS GRADUALLY

In post-surgery nutrition, the progressive introduction of solid foods represents a major turning point. In this phase, a greater range of foods, such as fruits, vegetables, and lean proteins, are reintroduced to the diet. The focus is on adding nutrient-dense foods that support healing and supply the building blocks required for the body to restore itself.

Tolerance to solid foods might vary from person to person, so it's important to pay attention to your body's signals and go at a comfortable speed for you.

FOODS TO ADD

A balanced approach is crucial when it comes to the meals that should be included in the post-surgery diet. Fish, poultry, and tofu are examples of lean proteins that aid in tissue healing and muscle strength restoration. Including a choice of vibrant fruits and vegetables guarantees a varied spectrum of vitamins, minerals, and antioxidants, all of which are essential for the healing process. While dairy products or dairy substitutes contribute to the consumption of calcium, which supports bone health during recovery, whole grains and complex carbs offer sustained energy.

ITEMS TO STEER CLEAR OF

On the other hand, there are several foods that you should stay away from after surgery. Fried foods, foods with a lot of added sugar, and highly processed foods can all cause inflammation and slow down the healing process. Since they may affect hydration levels and interfere with medication, caffeine, and alcohol should be used in moderation. To avoid straining the surgical site, people may also need to exercise caution while consuming meals that are hard to chew or digest, like fibrous vegetables or tough meats.

It should be noted that post-surgery nutrition guidelines cover a range of periods, from the initial postoperative period to the phased return of solid foods. These recommendations are meant to minimize risks while supplying vital nutrients to aid in the body's healing process. Maintaining a healthy diet that includes fruits, vegetables, lean meats, and other well-balanced foods as well as avoiding particular foods is essential for a speedy recovery and the enhancement of general well-being.

CHAPTER SIX

EXAMPLE MENUS

A CALM OVERVIEW OF SOLID FOODS

A baby's introduction to solid meals is a critical developmental milestone that signifies the change from just breastfeeding or formula feeding to a more varied diet. Around six months of age, when the baby can sit up with assistance, shows curiosity in the food that other people are eating and has sufficient head and neck control, this procedure is usually started. With the knowledge that every infant is different and may react differently to the introduction of solids, it's crucial to handle this transition with care.

To keep things familiar, start your trip with single-grain infant cereals like rice or oatmeal combined with breast milk or formula. Babies are assisted in acclimating to the new textures by gradually moving from a liquid to a thicker consistency. After that, add pureed fruits and veggies one at a time, giving the food at least three to five days to settle before adding another. This method facilitates a seamless transition to a more diversified diet while assisting in the identification of any possible allergies or sensitivities.

A STEP-BY-STEP GUIDE TO A BALANCED DIET

It's critical to move toward a balanced diet that includes a range of nutrients as babies develop and get more acclimated to eating solid meals. Add well-cooked and finely shredded meats, as well as mashed or finely chopped soft fruits and vegetables, at about the seven to eight-month mark. Introducing various flavors and textures helps the development of swallowing and chewing abilities.

Continue to increase the range of foods supplied after nine to twelve months. To promote self-feeding, offer modest servings of dairy products like cheese or yogurt and soft finger foods. Introduce a greater variety of grains and alternative protein sources, such as lentils and beans, gradually.

To promote ideal growth and development, it's critical to keep the ratios of healthy fats, proteins, and carbs in check.

WEEKS 5 AND UP SUSTAINING A DIET HIGH IN NUTRIENTS

Maintaining a nutrient-rich diet that promotes the infant's general health and development becomes more important as they approach the fifth week of solid food introduction and beyond. At this point, the infant ought to should be able to eat a wide variety of meals and feel at ease with a range of textures.

Incorporate a variety of complete grains, fruits, vegetables, proteins, and healthy fats into their regular meals. To guarantee a wide range of vitamins and minerals, serve a rainbow of fruits and vegetables. As you continue to introduce new meals, observe the baby's dietary preferences and any sensitivity.

To satisfy their expanding nutritional needs as the baby gets closer to the first year of life, think about including whole cow's milk and other dairy products along with a range of protein sources.

 The ultimate objective is to create lifelong healthy eating habits at a young age, laying the groundwork for a balanced diet. To guarantee a healthy and pleasurable eating experience, periodically evaluate the baby's growth, development, and nutritional preferences and modify the meal plan accordingly.

CHAPTER SEVEN

INCLUDING ADDENDA

SUPPLEMENTS' PLACE IN RECOVERY

The use of supplements in rehabilitation has drawn a lot of attention in the field of health and wellness, and it is now a crucial part of many people's daily regimens. Supplements are essential for assisting the body's recuperation, particularly following physically demanding activities or during times of heightened demand. To supply vital elements that may be absent from regular meals, these supplements are meant to be used in conjunction with a balanced diet.

SUGGESTED ADD-ONS

Omega-3 fatty acids are one of the supplements advised to aid in the healing process. These vital fats are well known for their anti-inflammatory qualities, which are crucial in lessening joint stiffness and muscle discomfort. Omega-3s, which are frequently present in fish oil supplements, support soft tissue healing and general joint health. Adding Omega-3 fatty acids to your diet can be especially helpful for people who are healing from injuries or participating in strenuous physical activity.

D-VITAMIN

Another essential supplement that is crucial to the healing process is vitamin D. Vitamin D, sometimes known as the "sunshine vitamin," is crucial for strong bones, a healthy immune system, and general well-being. Sustaining adequate levels of Vitamin D during the healing process is essential because it facilitates the body's absorption of calcium and builds bone mass. Sufficient consumption of Vitamin D is particularly important for people who don't get much sun exposure or are healing from bone-related ailments.

SUPPLEMENTS OF PROTEIN

It is often acknowledged that protein supplements play a crucial role in aiding in the healing process, especially for those participating in physically demanding activities like strength or endurance training. Since protein is the building block of muscle, adding protein to your diet with shakes or powders can help with both muscle growth and repair. For example, whey protein is a well-liked option because of its quick absorption and high amino acid content, which promote effective muscle synthesis and recovery.

It is important to recognize that every person's demands are different when it comes to recommended vitamins for recuperation. Personalized advice based on particular medical conditions, nutritional preferences, and exercise objectives can be obtained by speaking with nutritionists or healthcare specialists. Furthermore, it's still critical to keep a diet rich in nutrients and well-rounded, with supplements acting as supplemental means of filling in any nutritional gaps.

Adding supplements to your recovery regimen is a calculated move that will improve your body's capacity to heal and recover. Protein supplements, vitamin D, and omega-3 fatty acids are just a few of the numerous options available to promote various elements of the healing process. Together with a healthy diet and regular exercise, a well-considered and customized supplement regimen can greatly enhance general well-being and hasten recovery.

CHAPTER EIGHT

MAINTAINING HYDRATION

THE BENEFITS OF HYDRATION FOR HEALING

Maintaining proper hydration is essential for general health and is especially important throughout the healing process. To ensure optimal function of the body, it is imperative to maintain appropriate amounts of hydration, even after recovering from severe physical activity, illness, or injury. Dehydration can have a detrimental effect on several physiological functions in the body, making it more difficult for the body to mend and recover properly.

Sufficient hydration is critical during the healing process for several reasons. First of all, water is an essential component of numerous bodily biological events. Water is a medium for a variety of functions, including metabolic and cellular repair. Adequate hydration enables the body to heal injured tissues more efficiently, resulting in a quicker and more seamless recuperation.

Furthermore, the body's capacity to control its temperature is intimately related to hydration. The body may suffer temperature changes during recovery as it attempts to mend and heal itself. Maintaining an ideal body temperature through proper hydration allows the body to perform its healing processes effectively and stress-free.

SUGGESTED FLUID CONSUMPTION

Variations exist in the required fluid consumption according to age, sex, climate, and degree of activity. Still, it's generally recommended to drink eight 8-ounce glasses of water or more each day—a practice known as the "8x8 rule." This is roughly equivalent to two liters or half a gallon. It's crucial to remember that each person may have different demands for hydration and that when calculating fluid requirements, variables like physical activity, the weather, and general health should be taken into account.

Athletes and those who exercise vigorously might need to drink more fluids to make up for the extra fluids they lose via perspiration. In these situations, a customized strategy for hydration is essential, taking into account individual sweat rates as well as the length and intensity of the exercise. Sports drinks or electrolyte-rich beverages may also help replenish vital minerals lost after extended physical activity.

FOODS THAT HYDRATE

Although the main source of hydration is water, it's important to remember that foods high in water content can make a big difference in how much fluid is consumed overall. Particularly fruits and vegetables are high in water content and might be beneficial additions to a diet. Citrus fruits, celery, cucumbers, watermelon, and oranges are hydrating foods that help fulfill daily fluid needs while also offering vital nutrients. A delightful and efficient method to stay hydrated is to include a range of these items in your diet, especially if you struggle to get enough fluids from drinks alone.

It is impossible to overestimate the role that water plays in the healing process. Adequate consumption of fluids is essential for maintaining the body's biochemical functions, controlling body temperature, and promoting general healing processes. Maintaining ideal hydration levels for enhanced recuperation and well-being requires knowing one's own hydration needs, including hydrating foods in the diet, and being aware of variables affecting fluid requirements.

CHAPTER NINE

OVERCOMING OBSTACLES IN DIET

HANDLING DIGESTIVE PROBLEMS

One of the main obstacles people have while trying to keep a healthy diet is dealing with digestive problems. These issues can vary in severity from minor discomfort to more serious ailments like inflammatory bowel disorders (IBD) or irritable bowel syndrome (IBS).

It is critical to recognize trigger meals that may intensify digestive problems to overcome these difficulties. Maintaining a food journal and gradually removing possible offenders can assist in identifying particular triggers and enable the creation of a customized eating plan. Including foods that are simple to digest, like lean proteins and steamed veggies can frequently help. Additionally, you can improve digestion and lessen discomfort by drinking plenty of water and eating mindfully, which involves chewing your food properly.

HANDLING DIETARY LIMITS

Whether brought on by allergies, intolerances, or certain medical problems, dietary limits pose special difficulties that need to be carefully considered. Food allergy sufferers need to carefully examine ingredient lists and labels to steer clear of any possible allergens. Those who have intolerances, such as gluten sensitivity or lactose intolerance, must look for appropriate replacements and alternatives. Despite limitations, adopting a varied and well-balanced diet is crucial to guaranteeing sufficient nutrient intake. Experimenting and learning about different grains, plant-based proteins, and dairy substitutes can yield solutions that balance nutrients and adhere to dietary limitations.

SEEKING EXPERT NUTRITIONAL GUIDANCE

Consulting a nutritionist's knowledge is often necessary while navigating the complicated terrain of dietary problems. Nutritionists or registered dietitians can provide tailored advice based on each person's particular goals, dietary preferences, and state of health. These experts can assist in developing a personalized meal plan that takes into account dietary constraints or digestive problems while satisfying particular nutritional requirements.

Getting expert nutritional advice gives people the knowledge and tools they need to make wise food decisions in addition to offering an organized approach to diet management. Frequent meetings with a nutrition specialist can also be used to monitor development, make required modifications, and provide continuing assistance in the pursuit of ideal health.

Overcoming dietary obstacles requires a comprehensive strategy that takes into account unique requirements and situations. Incorporating easily digestible options and carefully examining trigger meals are necessary for managing digestive difficulties.

Dietary constraints necessitate imaginative food selection, attentive label reading, and a dedication to preserving nutritional equilibrium.

Getting expert nutritional advice guarantees a customized approach to diet management and provides insightful information and encouragement in the quest for a sustainable and healthy way of life.

CHAPTER TEN

EXERCISE AND RECOVERY

EXERCISE INTRODUCED GRADUALLY

A crucial part of physical activity and rehabilitation is the gradual introduction of exercise. This idea recognizes that introducing physical activities into a person's routine—especially for those undergoing rehabilitation—requires a methodical and incremental approach.

Exercises should be introduced gradually to allow the body to strengthen and adapt without risk of further injury, whether the goal is treating a chronic disease, healing from surgery, or recuperating from an injury. This approach takes into account the person's initial level of fitness, making sure that the workout program fits their skills and advances at a rate that encourages safe and long-lasting gains.

INCLUDING PHYSICAL THERAPY

The idea of incorporating physical therapy into rehabilitation is essential and emphasizes the value of a multidisciplinary approach. With their specialized training and abilities, physical therapists work with patients to create personalized exercise regimens that target particular rehabilitation objectives. These programs include a range of manual techniques, modalities, and therapeutic exercises designed to improve strength, flexibility, and mobility. Physical therapy integration not only speeds up the healing process but also gives people the confidence to take an active role in their rehabilitation, encouraging a sense of responsibility and dedication to the healing process.

TRACKING DEVELOPMENT

Any rehabilitation program must include progress monitoring as a crucial component, highlighting the necessity of ongoing evaluation and modification. Healthcare providers can assess the efficacy of the selected exercises, pinpoint areas for development, and adjust the rehabilitation plan based on ongoing review. Tracking functional abilities, pain thresholds, and physical gains are all part of the progress monitoring process.

Healthcare professionals may make well-informed decisions thanks to this data-driven approach, which guarantees that the rehabilitation program changes to meet the needs of the individual as they change. Frequent evaluations also promote candid communication between the patient and their medical team, creating a cooperative and encouraging atmosphere that is ideal for a full recovery.

The notions of introducing exercise gradually, incorporating physical therapy, and keeping track of progress are intricate components within the field of physical activity and rehabilitation. Through the implementation of a methodical and incremental exercise regimen, customization of physical therapy techniques, and regular progress tracking, healthcare practitioners can enhance rehabilitation results, enabling patients to regain functionality and enhance their general state of health. These ideas highlight how crucial customized and flexible rehabilitation plans are on the path to physical healing.

CHAPTER ELEVEN

LONG-TERM NUTRITIONAL FACTORS

SUSTAINING A HEALTHY LIFESTYLE

Sustaining a healthy lifestyle entails taking a comprehensive strategy that takes into account many facets of well-being, such as dietary decisions, exercise, stress reduction, and enough sleep.

A healthy, well-balanced diet is essential for maintaining general health. Eating a range of nutrient-dense foods, including whole grains, fruits, vegetables, lean meats, and healthy fats, must be prioritized. Staying properly hydrated is equally important since water facilitates several body processes and helps with nutrient absorption and digestion.

An additional essential component of a healthy lifestyle is regular physical activity. Combining aerobic, strength, and flexibility training improves cardiovascular health and further supports overall well-being by helping one maintain a healthy weight.

Furthermore, reducing stress through hobbies, mindfulness, or meditation can have a substantial positive impact on long-term health. Sufficient and high-quality sleep plays a crucial role in the body's recuperation and upkeep, influencing immune response, cognitive abilities, and general health.

NUTRITION FOR HEALTHY JOINTS

As people age, their joints become increasingly important to their long-term health. To support and maintain healthy joints, nutrition is essential. Walnuts, flaxseeds, and fish oil are good sources of omega-3 fatty acids, which have anti-inflammatory qualities that can help reduce stiffness and soreness in the joints. Rich in collagen found in bone broth and some supplements, collagen promotes joint structure and may help to enhance joint function.

Minerals and vitamins including calcium, vitamin D, and vitamin C are necessary for strong bones and can help fend against diseases like osteoporosis. Fruits and vegetables are rich in antioxidants, which help to prevent oxidative stress and inflammation that can harm joint structures. It's also critical to maintain a healthy weight because being overweight puts extra strain on joints, especially the knees and hips, which bear the brunt of the body's weight.

TECHNIQUES TO AVOID FUTURE ACCIDENTS

Future injury prevention calls for a diversified strategy that incorporates both preventive and reactive actions. Exercises for conditioning and strength training can increase muscle strength and flexibility while lowering the chance of injury. To prepare the body and aid in recovery, pay close attention to appropriate warm-up and cool-down exercises before and after physical activity.

To avoid straining joints and muscles, it is crucial to maintain appropriate biomechanics throughout workouts and daily activities. Important elements of injury prevention include paying attention to your body's signals, avoiding overtraining, and scheduling rest days into your training schedule.

Reducing the risk of cramps and muscular strains is possible by maintaining adequate hydration, which also improves overall physiological function and joint lubrication.

Frequent screenings and examinations of the health might reveal prospective risk factors or current conditions that may make people more vulnerable to injury. Seeking expert assistance, such as from physical therapy or sports medicine, can offer individualized plans to address particular deficiencies or imbalances in the body, reducing the likelihood of further injuries. Maintaining long-term physical health and well-being is facilitated by implementing these preventive practices into daily living.